Optimal Nutrition:

Fueling Your Body for Peak Performance

By

Mary F. Scott

TABLE OF CONTENTS

CHAPTER I
Introduction

A. Importance of nutrition in achieving peak performance

Nutrition plays a paramount role in achieving peak performance. Whether you are an athlete, a fitness enthusiast, or simply someone striving to reach your full potential, fueling your body with optimal nutrition is essential. The food we consume acts as the foundation for our physical and mental well-being, directly influencing our energy levels, focus, endurance, and overall performance.

The human body is a remarkable machine, capable of incredible feats. However, like any machine, it requires the right fuel to operate at its best. Just as a high-performance car needs premium gasoline to achieve maximum speed and efficiency, our bodies require a well-balanced and nourishing diet to function optimally. Without proper nutrition, our performance potential remains untapped, and we may experience fatigue, reduced stamina, impaired recovery, and decreased cognitive function.

When we talk about peak performance, it encompasses various aspects of life. It extends beyond the realm of professional athletes and spills into everyday activities, such as excelling at work, maintaining focus during studies, or simply engaging in recreational activities with vigor and vitality. Nutrition acts as a catalyst for reaching new heights in all these areas.

The impact of nutrition on performance is multifaceted. Macronutrients like carbohydrates, proteins, and fats provide the necessary energy for physical activities and ensure proper muscle function. They serve as the building blocks for repairing and building new tissues, promoting strength and endurance. Additionally, micronutrients such as vitamins and minerals act as co-factors in countless metabolic processes, influencing energy production, immune function, and cognitive abilities.

By understanding our nutritional needs and tailoring our dietary choices accordingly, we can unlock our true potential. This book, "Optimal Nutrition: Fueling Your Body for Peak Performance," serves as a comprehensive guide to help you navigate the intricate world of nutrition and make informed choices that will propel you towards success. Whether you are an athlete striving for athletic greatness or an individual seeking to enhance your daily performance, this book will equip you with the knowledge and strategies necessary to optimize your nutrition.

Throughout the chapters, we will delve into the fundamental principles of nutrition, dissecting macronutrients and micronutrients, exploring the intricacies of timing and composition of meals, and providing practical strategies to overcome common nutritional challenges. We will also examine how nutrition varies across different sports and activities, as well as the potential role of supplementation in enhancing performance.

It's time to unleash your full potential and unlock the power of nutrition. Together, let us embark on a journey towards achieving peak performance by fueling your body with optimal nutrition. By the end of this book, you will have the tools and insights to revolutionize your approach to food, enhance your performance, and embrace a healthier, more vibrant lifestyle. Get ready to take the first step towards a stronger, fitter, and more fulfilled you.

B. Overview of the book's purpose and content

In this fast-paced world where performance and productivity are highly valued, it has become increasingly important to understand the vital role that nutrition plays in fueling our bodies for peak performance. This book, "Optimal Nutrition: Fueling Your Body for Peak Performance," aims to provide a comprehensive guide to help you harness the power of nutrition and optimize your physical and mental capabilities.

The purpose of this book is to offer a roadmap that leads you through the intricate realm of nutrition, offering valuable insights, evidence-based information, and practical strategies to achieve optimal performance. Whether you are an athlete striving for excellence, a professional seeking to enhance your cognitive abilities, or simply someone yearning to live a healthier and more vibrant life, this book is designed to cater to your unique needs.

Throughout the pages of this book, we will explore a wide range of topics, beginning with an understanding of nutrition's fundamental principles. We will unravel the science behind macronutrients and micronutrients, explaining how carbohydrates, proteins, and fats serve as the building blocks for energy, muscle repair, and overall vitality. We will delve into the world of vitamins and minerals, uncovering their critical roles in metabolic processes and immune function.

Assessing your individual nutritional needs is a crucial step on the path to optimal performance, and this book will guide you through the process. We will help you determine your caloric requirements based on your activity levels, goals, and body composition. Additionally, we will explore the specific nutrient needs for different types of activities, ensuring that you are equipped with the knowledge to fuel your body in the most effective way.

Designing a well-balanced meal plan is essential for meeting your nutritional goals, and we will provide practical strategies for achieving this. From understanding portion sizes to incorporating nutrient-dense foods into your diet, you will learn how to create meals that not only fuel your body but also promote long-term health and vitality.

Pre-performance and post-performance nutrition strategies are key elements in maximizing your potential. We will uncover the importance of fueling your body before workouts or competitions, discussing the optimal timing and composition of pre-workout meals. We will also explore the critical role of recovery nutrition, emphasizing the replenishment of glycogen stores, muscle repair, and rehydration to enhance your body's ability to bounce back after exertion.

Furthermore, we will address the specific nutritional considerations for different sports and activities. Whether you are an endurance athlete, a strength trainer, or a team sports enthusiast, this book will provide tailored insights and strategies to optimize your nutrition for your chosen field.

Supplementation is a topic that often sparks curiosity and controversy. We will take an objective approach, exploring the role of supplements in performance enhancement. You will gain an understanding of commonly used supplements, their potential benefits, and the associated risks. We will emphasize responsible supplementation, empowering you to make informed decisions about whether and how to incorporate supplements into your nutritional regimen.

Overcoming common nutritional challenges is another aspect that we will tackle in this book. From dealing with dietary restrictions and allergies to navigating dining out or traveling, we will provide practical tips and solutions to help you maintain optimal nutrition in various situations.

Finally, we will delve into the significance of long-term nutrition and lifestyle habits. We will discuss the importance of sustainable eating practices, as well as the impact of sleep, stress management, and recovery on performance. By embracing a holistic approach to your well-being, you will be able to unlock your full potential and maintain peak performance in the long run.

Through "Optimal Nutrition: Fueling Your Body for Peak Performance," you will gain the knowledge, tools, and inspiration to transform your relationship with food and harness its incredible power to fuel your body and mind. Get ready to embark on an enlightening journey towards a healthier, more vibrant, and high-performing you.

CHAPTER II
Understanding Nutrition

A. Basics of Macronutrients and Micronutrients

When it comes to optimizing nutrition for peak performance, it is crucial to have a solid understanding of macronutrients and micronutrients. These essential components of our diet play distinct roles in fueling and nourishing our bodies.

Macronutrients are the three main categories of nutrients that provide energy: carbohydrates, proteins, and fats. Carbohydrates are the primary source of energy for the body, supplying fuel for both physical activities and brain function. They come in two forms: simple carbohydrates, found in foods like fruits and sugary snacks, and complex carbohydrates, which are found in whole grains, legumes, and vegetables. Balancing carbohydrate intake is vital to maintain steady energy levels and sustain physical performance.

Proteins are essential for repairing and building tissues, including muscles, tendons, and organs. They are composed of amino acids, which act as the building blocks for various cellular functions. Good sources of protein include lean meats, poultry, fish, dairy products, legumes, and nuts. Athletes and individuals engaged in regular physical activity may require higher protein intake to support muscle repair and growth.

Fats, often misunderstood, are an important energy source and play a critical role in hormone production, nutrient absorption, and insulation of vital organs. They can be divided into unsaturated fats (found in nuts, avocados, and vegetable oils) and saturated fats (found in animal products and some processed foods). It is essential to choose healthy sources of fats and strike a balance in their consumption for optimal health and performance.

Micronutrients, on the other hand, are essential vitamins and minerals required in smaller quantities but are no less important. Vitamins are organic compounds that aid in various physiological processes, such as energy metabolism and immune function. They can be categorized into water-soluble vitamins (like vitamin C and B-complex vitamins) and fat-soluble vitamins (like vitamins A, D, E, and K), each with specific roles and sources.

Minerals are inorganic elements that contribute to many bodily functions, such as bone health, nerve function, and fluid balance. Examples of minerals include calcium, iron, zinc, magnesium, and potassium, which can be obtained from a variety of food sources.

Understanding the balance and importance of macronutrients and micronutrients is the first step in optimizing nutrition for peak performance. By incorporating a variety of nutrient-rich foods into our diet, we can ensure that we provide our bodies with the necessary fuel and building blocks to perform at our best.

In the following chapters, we will delve deeper into the functions, recommended intake, and food sources of macronutrients and micronutrients. By gaining a comprehensive understanding of these nutritional components, you will be empowered to make informed choices about your diet and fuel your body in a way that enhances your performance and overall well-being.

B. Exploring the Role of Carbohydrates, Proteins, and Fats in the Body

Carbohydrates, proteins, and fats are the three macronutrients that play vital roles in the functioning of our bodies. Each of these nutrients serves distinct purposes and provides energy in different ways, contributing to our overall health and performance.

Carbohydrates are the body's primary source of energy. When consumed, carbohydrates are broken down into glucose, which is then used as fuel for various bodily functions. Glucose is not only important for physical activities but also plays a crucial role in brain function. Carbohydrates can be found in foods such as grains, fruits, vegetables, and legumes. Simple carbohydrates, like those found in sugar and processed foods, provide quick bursts of energy, while complex carbohydrates, found in whole grains and starchy vegetables, provide sustained energy over a longer period. It is important to choose carbohydrates wisely and consume them in appropriate portions to maintain stable energy levels and support optimal performance.

Proteins are essential for the growth, repair, and maintenance of tissues in the body. They are made up of amino acids, which are the building blocks of protein. During digestion, proteins are broken down into amino acids, which are then utilized by the body for various purposes. Adequate protein intake is particularly important for athletes and individuals engaging in regular physical activity, as it supports muscle repair and growth. Good sources of protein include lean meats, poultry, fish, eggs, dairy products, legumes, and plant-based sources such as tofu and quinoa.

Fats, often misconceived as being unhealthy, are an important macronutrient that plays several vital roles in the body. They are a concentrated source of energy and help in the absorption of fat-soluble vitamins. Fats also provide insulation and protection for organs, aid in hormone production, and contribute to cell structure.

Healthy fats, such as monounsaturated and polyunsaturated fats found in foods like avocados, nuts, seeds, and fatty fish, are beneficial for cardiovascular health and overall well-being. It is important to moderate saturated and trans fats, found in high amounts in processed and fried foods, as they can negatively impact health if consumed excessively.

The role of carbohydrates, proteins, and fats in the body goes beyond energy provision. They are intricately involved in various physiological processes, including enzyme production, hormone regulation, immune function, and cell signaling. Each macronutrient has its own specific functions, but they also work together synergistically to support overall health and performance.

In the subsequent chapters, we will delve deeper into the specific functions and optimal intake of carbohydrates, proteins, and fats. You will gain insights into the importance of each macronutrient, discover how to incorporate them into your diet in appropriate proportions, and learn how to optimize their consumption for peak performance. By understanding the distinct roles and benefits of carbohydrates, proteins, and fats, you will be empowered to make informed choices and create a well-balanced diet that fuels your body and supports your performance goals.

C. Understanding Vitamins, Minerals, and Their Functions

Vitamins and minerals, often referred to as micronutrients, are essential components of our diet that play critical roles in supporting various bodily functions. While they are required in smaller quantities compared to macronutrients, their importance cannot be overstated. Let's explore the world of vitamins, minerals, and their functions in the body.

Vitamins are organic compounds that are necessary for the proper functioning of our bodies. They are classified into two categories: water-soluble vitamins and fat-soluble vitamins. Water-soluble vitamins include vitamin C and the B-complex vitamins, such as B1 (thiamine), B2 (riboflavin), B3 (niacin), B6 (pyridoxine), B9 (folate), and B12 (cobalamin). These vitamins are not stored in the body and need to be consumed regularly as they are easily excreted. They are involved in a wide range of functions, including energy metabolism, immune support, and nerve function.

On the other hand, fat-soluble vitamins, including vitamins A, D, E, and K, are stored in the body's fat tissues and liver. They require fat for absorption and can be stored for longer periods. Vitamin A is essential for vision, immune function, and cell growth. Vitamin D plays a crucial role in bone health and calcium absorption. Vitamin E acts as an antioxidant, protecting cells from damage. Vitamin K is involved in blood clotting and bone metabolism.

Minerals, like vitamins, are vital for maintaining optimal health and well-being. They are inorganic substances that are necessary for various physiological processes. Some essential minerals include calcium, iron, zinc, magnesium, potassium, and sodium.

Calcium is crucial for bone health, muscle function, and nerve transmission. Iron is essential for the production of red blood cells and oxygen transport. Zinc plays a role in immune function, wound healing, and protein synthesis. Magnesium is involved in hundreds of biochemical reactions in the body, including energy production and muscle relaxation. Potassium and sodium are electrolytes that help maintain fluid balance, nerve function, and muscle contractions.

Each vitamin and mineral serves a specific purpose in the body, and their deficiency or excess can have significant impacts on our health and performance. Consuming a varied and balanced diet that includes a wide range of fruits, vegetables, whole grains, lean proteins, and dairy products can help ensure an adequate intake of these essential micronutrients.

In the upcoming chapters, we will delve deeper into the functions and food sources of vitamins and minerals. You will gain a comprehensive understanding of how these micronutrients contribute to overall health and performance, and learn strategies to optimize their intake. By harnessing the power of vitamins and minerals, you will be able to support your body's physiological processes, enhance your immunity, and optimize your performance potential.

CHAPTER III
Assessing Your Nutritional Needs

A. Determining Your Caloric Requirements

Understanding your caloric requirements is an essential step in optimizing your nutrition for peak performance. Calories serve as the measure of energy obtained from food, and finding the right balance is crucial for maintaining a healthy weight and supporting your physical and mental activities.

Several factors influence your caloric needs, including your age, gender, weight, height, activity level, and goals. There are various methods to estimate your daily caloric requirements, and one commonly used approach is the Harris-Benedict equation. This equation takes into account your basal metabolic rate (BMR), which is the amount of energy your body needs to perform basic functions at rest, and applies an activity factor to calculate your total daily energy expenditure (TDEE).

To determine your caloric needs, you can start by calculating your BMR. The Harris-Benedict equation provides separate formulas for males and females:

For males: BMR = 88.362 + (13.397 × weight in kg) + (4.799 × height in cm) - (5.677 × age in years)

For females: BMR = 447.593 + (9.247 × weight in kg) + (3.098 × height in cm) - (4.330 × age in years)

After obtaining your BMR, you need to apply an activity factor to estimate your TDEE. The activity factor accounts for the calories burned through physical activity. Here are some common activity factors:

- Sedentary (little to no exercise): BMR × 1.2

- Lightly active (light exercise/sports 1-3 days a week): BMR × 1.375

- Moderately active (moderate exercise/sports 3-5 days a week): BMR × 1.55

- Very active (hard exercise/sports 6-7 days a week): BMR × 1.725

- Extra active (very hard exercise/sports and physical job or training twice a day): BMR × 1.9

Once you have calculated your TDEE, you can adjust your caloric intake based on your goals. To maintain your current weight, you would aim to consume approximately the same number of calories as your TDEE. To lose weight, you would create a calorie deficit by consuming fewer calories, typically around 500-1000 calories less than your TDEE per day. Conversely, to gain weight, you would aim for a calorie surplus by consuming more calories than your TDEE.

It's important to note that these calculations provide rough estimates, and individual variations can occur. Factors such as metabolism, body composition, and overall health can influence your caloric needs. Consulting with a registered dietitian or nutritionist can provide personalized guidance in determining your specific requirements.

In the following chapters, we will explore strategies to fine-tune your nutrient intake based on your caloric needs and performance goals. By understanding and meeting your caloric requirements, you will ensure that your body receives the energy it needs to thrive, supporting your physical performance, mental acuity, and overall well-being.

B. Analyzing Individual Dietary Goals and Activity Levels

When it comes to optimizing nutrition for peak performance, it's important to analyze your individual dietary goals and activity levels. Tailoring your nutritional approach to your specific needs will help you achieve optimal results and enhance your overall performance.

Dietary Goals:

Analyzing your dietary goals is a crucial step in assessing your nutritional needs. Whether your goal is to improve athletic performance, lose weight, gain muscle, or simply maintain a healthy lifestyle, your dietary choices should align with those objectives.

For athletes or individuals engaged in intense physical activity, fueling the body with adequate energy and nutrients is essential. This may involve adjusting macronutrient ratios, increasing overall caloric intake, and focusing on nutrient timing to optimize energy levels and recovery.

If weight loss is your goal, it's important to create a calorie deficit by consuming fewer calories than your body requires. This can be achieved by selecting nutrient-dense, low-calorie foods, managing portion sizes, and incorporating regular physical activity into your routine.

For those aiming to build muscle or enhance strength, a focus on protein intake becomes crucial. Consuming an adequate amount of high-quality protein supports muscle repair and growth, while also ensuring overall nutrient balance.

Activity Levels:

Analyzing your activity levels is another important factor in assessing your nutritional needs. The energy demands of your physical activities play a significant role in determining the amount of calories and nutrients you require.

Individuals with a sedentary lifestyle or minimal physical activity may have lower caloric needs compared to those who engage in regular exercise or have physically demanding jobs. In contrast, athletes and individuals involved in intense training or endurance activities will likely require higher caloric intake to fuel their performance and aid in recovery.

Analyzing your activity levels helps in determining the appropriate macronutrient distribution and overall caloric intake needed to support your energy requirements and optimize performance.

By carefully analyzing your dietary goals and activity levels, you can create a personalized nutrition plan that addresses your specific needs. Consulting with a registered dietitian or nutritionist can provide valuable guidance in assessing your goals and designing an individualized approach.

In the upcoming chapters, we will delve deeper into strategies for analyzing and fine-tuning your dietary goals and activity levels. You will gain insights into the importance of macronutrient distribution, nutrient timing, and the role of supplements in supporting your individual needs. By understanding and analyzing your dietary goals and activity levels, you will be equipped with the knowledge and tools to design a nutrition plan that fuels your body, enhances your performance, and helps you achieve your desired outcomes.

C. Assessing Specific Nutrient Needs for Optimal Performance

To achieve optimal performance, it is essential to assess your specific nutrient needs. While macronutrients (carbohydrates, proteins, and fats) form the foundation of your diet, other micronutrients and key compounds also play crucial roles in supporting your body's functions and enhancing performance.

Micronutrients:

Micronutrients, including vitamins and minerals, are essential for various physiological processes. Assessing your specific micronutrient needs involves identifying any potential deficiencies or areas where additional support may be required.

Vitamins such as vitamin C, vitamin E, and the B-complex vitamins contribute to energy production, immune function, and cellular health. Minerals like iron, calcium, magnesium, and zinc are involved in muscle function, bone health, and metabolism.

Analyzing your dietary intake and considering factors such as age, gender, activity level, and specific health conditions can help identify any micronutrient gaps and guide adjustments to your diet or supplementation as needed.

Hydration:

Hydration is a critical aspect of optimal performance. Assessing your hydration needs involves understanding the demands placed on your body and maintaining proper fluid balance.

Factors such as climate, activity level, duration and intensity of exercise, and individual sweat rates impact your fluid requirements. Adequate hydration supports thermoregulation, nutrient transport, and overall cellular function.

Monitoring your fluid intake and paying attention to thirst cues can help you maintain optimal hydration levels. Adjusting your fluid intake based on environmental conditions and the intensity of your activities is crucial for optimal performance.

Key Compounds:

In addition to macronutrients and micronutrients, certain key compounds can positively impact performance. These include antioxidants, omega-3 fatty acids, and dietary fiber.

Antioxidants, found in fruits, vegetables, and nuts, help combat oxidative stress and inflammation in the body. Omega-3 fatty acids, abundant in fatty fish, flaxseeds, and walnuts, have anti-inflammatory properties and support cardiovascular health and brain function. Dietary fiber, obtained from whole grains, fruits, and vegetables, aids digestion, regulates blood sugar levels, and promotes satiety.

Assessing your intake of these key compounds and adjusting your diet to incorporate adequate amounts can contribute to optimal performance and overall well-being.

By assessing your specific nutrient needs, you can fine-tune your diet to optimize performance. Incorporating a variety of nutrient-rich foods, considering supplementation when necessary, and staying properly hydrated will support your body's demands and help you reach peak performance.

In the following chapters, we will explore strategies for assessing and meeting specific nutrient needs. You will gain insights into optimizing micronutrient intake, implementing hydration strategies, and incorporating key compounds into your diet.

CHAPTER IV
Designing a Balanced Meal Plan

A. The Concept of a Well-Balanced Diet

A well-balanced diet forms the foundation of optimal nutrition for peak performance. It involves consuming a variety of foods from different food groups to ensure an adequate intake of essential nutrients. The concept of a well-balanced diet focuses on achieving a harmonious combination of macronutrients, micronutrients, and other important components for overall health and performance.

Macronutrients:

Macronutrients, including carbohydrates, proteins, and fats, are the primary sources of energy in our diet. Each macronutrient plays a distinct role in supporting bodily functions and should be included in appropriate proportions in a well-balanced meal plan.

Carbohydrates provide the body with readily available energy and should make up a significant portion of your daily calorie intake. Opt for complex carbohydrates such as whole grains, fruits, and vegetables, which provide fiber and essential nutrients along with sustained energy.

Proteins are crucial for muscle repair, growth, and various physiological processes. Include lean sources of protein like poultry, fish, legumes, and dairy products to meet your daily protein needs.

Healthy fats, such as those found in avocados, nuts, seeds, and olive oil, are essential for hormone production, nutrient absorption, and brain function. Incorporate these sources of healthy fats into your meals while keeping portion sizes in mind.

Micronutrients:

Micronutrients, including vitamins and minerals, are vital for supporting overall health and performance. A well-balanced diet should encompass a variety of fruits, vegetables, whole grains, lean proteins, and dairy products to ensure an adequate intake of these essential nutrients.

Fruits and vegetables provide an array of vitamins, minerals, and antioxidants that support immune function, reduce inflammation, and promote overall well-being. Include a colorful assortment of fruits and vegetables in your meals to maximize the variety of micronutrients consumed.

Whole grains like quinoa, brown rice, and whole wheat bread offer essential vitamins, minerals, and fiber. These nutrients help regulate blood sugar levels, support digestion, and provide a steady release of energy.

Lean proteins, such as chicken, turkey, fish, and plant-based sources like tofu and legumes, provide a rich supply of essential amino acids and minerals. Aim to incorporate a variety of protein sources to ensure a well-rounded nutrient profile.

Dairy products like milk, yogurt, and cheese offer calcium, vitamin D, and other essential nutrients for bone health. If you have dietary restrictions or preferences, choose non-dairy alternatives that are fortified with essential nutrients.

Other Components:

In addition to macronutrients and micronutrients, other components contribute to a well-balanced diet. These include fiber, water, and phytochemicals.

Fiber, found in whole grains, fruits, vegetables, and legumes, aids digestion, promotes satiety, and supports heart health. Ensure an adequate intake of dietary fiber to maintain optimal digestive function.

Water is vital for hydration, nutrient transport, and overall cellular function. Make water your primary beverage choice and consume it throughout the day to stay adequately hydrated.

Phytochemicals, present in plant-based foods, have antioxidant and anti-inflammatory properties that contribute to overall health. Incorporate a diverse range of fruits, vegetables, herbs, and spices into your meals to maximize the intake of these beneficial compounds.

By understanding and embracing the concept of a well-balanced diet, you can design a meal plan that meets your nutritional needs and supports optimal performance. Focus on incorporating a variety of nutrient-dense foods, emphasizing whole grains, lean proteins, fruits, vegetables, healthy fats, and adequate hydration. Aim for moderation, portion control, and mindful eating practices to create a sustainable and enjoyable approach to fueling your body for peak performance.

In the upcoming chapters, we will delve deeper into designing and structuring a balanced meal plan that aligns with your goals and preferences. You will gain insights into meal timing, portion sizes, and strategies for maintaining a well-balanced diet while accommodating specific dietary needs. By implementing a well-balanced meal plan, you will set yourself up for success in achieving optimal nutrition and fueling your body for peak performance.

B. Planning Meals to Meet Macronutrient and Micronutrient Requirements

When designing a balanced meal plan, it is crucial to consider both macronutrient and micronutrient requirements. This ensures that you are fueling your body with the necessary nutrients for optimal performance and overall well-being. By strategically planning your meals, you can meet these requirements and create a nutritionally balanced eating pattern.

Macronutrient Requirements:

To meet your macronutrient requirements, focus on incorporating foods from each macronutrient group into your meals. Here are some guidelines for planning meals that address these needs:

a) Carbohydrates: Choose complex carbohydrates such as whole grains, legumes, and starchy vegetables. These provide a steady release of energy, fiber, and essential nutrients. Incorporate foods like quinoa, brown rice, sweet potatoes, and whole wheat bread into your meals to meet your carbohydrate needs.

b) Proteins: Include lean sources of protein to meet your protein requirements. Opt for skinless poultry, fish, lean cuts of meat, tofu, tempeh, and legumes. These sources provide essential amino acids for muscle repair and growth. Distribute your protein intake evenly across your meals to support optimal protein synthesis throughout the day.

c) Fats: Incorporate healthy fats into your meal plan. Avocados, nuts, seeds, olive oil, and fatty fish like salmon are excellent sources of omega-3 fatty acids and monounsaturated fats. These fats support brain function, hormone production, and overall health. Practice portion control as fats are calorie-dense.

Micronutrient Requirements:

Meeting your micronutrient requirements involves consuming a variety of nutrient-dense foods. Here are some strategies to ensure you're getting essential vitamins and minerals:

a) Fruits and Vegetables: Include a colorful assortment of fruits and vegetables in your meals to maximize your micronutrient intake. Different fruits and vegetables offer various vitamins, minerals, and antioxidants. Aim for a variety of colors to obtain a wide range of nutrients.

b) Whole Grains: Choose whole grains over refined grains to increase your intake of essential vitamins and minerals. Foods like whole wheat bread, oats, quinoa, and brown rice provide fiber, B vitamins, and minerals such as iron and magnesium.

c) Dairy or Alternatives: Include dairy products like milk, yogurt, and cheese to meet your calcium and vitamin D needs. If you have dietary restrictions or prefer non-dairy options, choose fortified alternatives like soy milk or almond milk.

d) Protein Sources: Select protein sources that provide additional micronutrients. For example, seafood like salmon and tuna are rich in omega-3 fatty acids, while spinach and legumes are good sources of iron. By choosing nutrient-dense protein sources, you can meet both macronutrient and micronutrient needs simultaneously.

Meal Planning Tips:

To effectively plan meals that meet your macronutrient and micronutrient requirements, consider these tips:

a) Create balanced meals by including a source of protein, carbohydrates, and healthy fats in each meal.

b) Emphasize whole, minimally processed foods to maximize nutrient content.

c) Prioritize nutrient-dense ingredients, such as leafy greens, berries, and lean proteins.

d) Plan your meals in advance to ensure variety and meet specific nutrient goals.

e) Use online resources or mobile apps to track your macronutrient and micronutrient intake.

f) Consider consulting with a registered dietitian or nutritionist for personalized guidance and support.

By planning meals that address both macronutrient and micronutrient requirements, you can ensure your body receives the necessary nutrients for optimal performance. Strive for balance, variety, and moderation in your meal plan to create a sustainable and nourishing approach to fueling your body for peak performance.

In the following chapters, we will explore practical meal planning strategies, portion control techniques, and recipe ideas to assist you in designing a balanced meal plan that meets your specific needs and enhances your performance.

C. Incorporating Nutrient-Dense Foods for Optimal Performance

When designing a balanced meal plan for optimal performance, it is crucial to prioritize nutrient-dense foods. Nutrient-dense foods are those that provide a high concentration of essential nutrients relative to their calorie content. By incorporating these foods into your meals, you can maximize your intake of vitamins, minerals, antioxidants, and other beneficial compounds that support overall health and performance.

Fruits and Vegetables:

Fruits and vegetables are nutritional powerhouses packed with vitamins, minerals, fiber, and antioxidants. They should form a significant portion of your meal plan. Aim to include a variety of colors to ensure a diverse range of nutrients.

Leafy greens like spinach, kale, and Swiss chard are excellent sources of vitamins A, C, K, and folate. Berries, such as blueberries, strawberries, and raspberries, are rich in antioxidants and provide a range of vitamins and minerals. Cruciferous vegetables like broccoli, cauliflower, and Brussels sprouts offer fiber, vitamin C, and other beneficial compounds.

Incorporate fruits and vegetables into your meals as salads, stir-fries, smoothies, or side dishes. Experiment with different cooking methods to retain their nutrient content.

Whole Grains:

Whole grains are an essential component of a balanced meal plan. They are rich in fiber, B vitamins, minerals, and phytochemicals. Opt for whole grain options such as quinoa, brown rice, oats, whole wheat bread, and whole grain pasta.

These nutrient-dense grains provide sustained energy and promote satiety. They also support digestion, regulate blood sugar levels, and contribute to heart health. Replace refined grains with whole grains in your meals to maximize nutrient intake.

Lean Proteins:

Incorporating lean proteins into your meal plan is crucial for muscle repair, growth, and overall performance. Choose lean sources such as skinless poultry, fish, lean cuts of meat, tofu, tempeh, and legumes.

Fish, especially fatty fish like salmon, mackerel, and sardines, provide omega-3 fatty acids that have anti-inflammatory properties and support brain health. Legumes like lentils, chickpeas, and black beans are excellent plant-based sources of protein, fiber, and various minerals.

Incorporate lean proteins into your meals as the main dish or as a component alongside grains and vegetables. Strive for a balance between animal and plant-based protein sources.

Healthy Fats:

Healthy fats are essential for optimal performance and overall health. They provide energy, support hormone production, aid nutrient absorption, and promote brain function. Incorporate nutrient-dense sources of healthy fats into your meals.

Avocados, nuts, seeds, olive oil, and fatty fish like salmon and trout are excellent choices. These foods offer monounsaturated fats, omega-3 fatty acids, and vitamin E. Practice portion control, as fats are calorie-dense.

Dairy or Alternatives:

Dairy products like milk, yogurt, and cheese provide calcium, protein, and other essential nutrients. If you have dietary restrictions or prefer non-dairy options, choose fortified alternatives like soy milk or almond milk.

Ensure these alternatives are fortified with calcium and vitamin D.

Consider incorporating low-fat or Greek yogurt into your meals as a protein-rich option. Use dairy or non-dairy alternatives in smoothies, cereal, or as a snack.

By prioritizing nutrient-dense foods in your meal plan, you can optimize your nutrient intake and support your body's performance needs. Aim for a balance of fruits, vegetables, whole grains, lean proteins, and healthy fats. Adapt your choices to accommodate specific dietary preferences or restrictions.

In the upcoming chapters, we will explore creative ways to incorporate these nutrient-dense foods into delicious and satisfying meals, providing you with practical strategies for optimizing your performance through nutrition.

CHAPTER V
Pre-Performance Nutrition Strategies

A. Fueling Your Body Before Workouts or Competitions

Fueling your body properly before workouts or competitions is essential for optimizing performance and ensuring sufficient energy levels. The pre-performance period is a critical time to provide your body with the right nutrients to enhance endurance, strength, focus, and overall performance. Consider the following strategies when planning your pre-performance nutrition:

Timing:

Timing your pre-performance meal is crucial to allow for proper digestion and absorption of nutrients. Aim to consume a meal or snack approximately 2-3 hours before your workout or competition. This timeframe allows enough time for digestion, preventing discomfort or side effects during physical activity.

Carbohydrates for Energy:

Prioritize carbohydrates as a primary fuel source during pre-performance nutrition. Complex carbohydrates, such as whole grains, fruits, and vegetables, provide a sustained release of energy and help maintain stable blood sugar levels. Include foods like oatmeal, quinoa, bananas, and sweet potatoes in your pre-performance meal to ensure an adequate carbohydrate intake.

Protein for Muscle Repair:

Including a moderate amount of protein in your pre-performance meal supports muscle repair and recovery. Opt for lean protein sources like chicken breast, turkey, fish, tofu, or Greek yogurt. These provide essential amino acids necessary for repairing and building muscle tissue.

Hydration:

Proper hydration is crucial before any physical activity. Ensure you are adequately hydrated by consuming fluids leading up to your workout or competition. Water is generally the best choice, but you may also consider incorporating electrolyte-rich beverages if you anticipate intense or prolonged exercise.

Meal Composition:

Design your pre-performance meal to be balanced and easily digestible. Include a combination of carbohydrates, protein, and a small amount of healthy fats. This combination provides sustained energy, promotes muscle repair, and helps maintain satiety.

Snack Options:

If your workout or competition is scheduled within an hour or two, choose lighter snack options to provide quick energy. Opt for easily digestible carbohydrates such as a piece of fruit, a granola bar, or a small smoothie. Consider including a small amount of protein for added satiety.

Personalization:

Tailor your pre-performance nutrition to your individual needs and preferences. Experiment with different food options and meal timing to determine what works best for you. Consider consulting with a sports nutritionist or registered dietitian for personalized guidance based on your specific goals and requirements.

Remember, consistency is key when it comes to pre-performance nutrition. Develop a routine that works for you and stick to it to optimize your energy levels, focus, and performance.

In the subsequent chapters, we will further explore pre-performance nutrition strategies, including specific meal and snack ideas, nutrient timing, and supplements that may enhance your performance before workouts or competitions.

B. Timing and Composition of Pre-Workout Meals

Timing and composition of pre-workout meals play a crucial role in providing your body with the necessary fuel and nutrients for optimal performance. By strategically planning your pre-workout meals, you can enhance energy levels, maximize endurance, and improve overall exercise performance. Consider the following guidelines when it comes to timing and composition:

Timing:

Timing your pre-workout meal is essential to ensure proper digestion and nutrient absorption. The ideal timing can vary depending on factors such as individual preferences, the intensity of the workout, and personal tolerance. However, a general guideline is to consume a meal or snack 1-3 hours before your workout.

- If you have 1-2 hours before your workout, opt for a light meal or substantial snack. This timeframe allows for digestion and minimizes the risk of discomfort during exercise.

- If you have 2-3 hours before your workout, you can consume a more substantial meal that includes a balance of carbohydrates, protein, and fats.

Carbohydrates:

Carbohydrates are the primary fuel source for exercise and are crucial for sustaining energy levels during your workout. Choose complex carbohydrates that provide a slow and steady release of energy. Some examples include whole grains, fruits, vegetables, and legumes.

Incorporate carbohydrate-rich foods into your pre-workout meal or snack. Oatmeal with berries, whole grain toast with nut butter, or a fruit and yogurt smoothie are excellent options. Aim to include around 30-60 grams of carbohydrates depending on the duration and intensity of your workout.

Protein:

Including protein in your pre-workout meal or snack can support muscle repair and recovery. It also helps to prevent muscle breakdown during exercise, particularly for longer and more intense workouts.

Opt for lean sources of protein such as chicken breast, fish, tofu, or Greek yogurt. Aim to include around 15-30 grams of protein in your pre-workout meal or snack.

Fats:

While fats provide a concentrated source of energy, it is recommended to keep fat intake relatively low in the pre-workout period. Higher fat meals can delay digestion and potentially cause discomfort during exercise.

However, incorporating small amounts of healthy fats, such as nuts, seeds, or avocado, can provide additional satiety and contribute to overall meal balance.

Fluids and Hydration:

Proper hydration is crucial for optimal performance. Make sure to hydrate adequately before your workout to prevent dehydration and maintain optimal body function. Consume water or a sports drink leading up to your workout depending on the duration and intensity of the exercise.

Individual Considerations:

Everyone's tolerance and preferences can vary when it comes to pre-workout nutrition. It is important to experiment and find what works best for you. Consider factors such as personal digestive tolerance, energy needs, and individual goals.

Pre-Workout Snacks:

If you have limited time before your workout, choose easily digestible, smaller snack options. Opt for a piece of fruit, a handful of nuts, or a protein bar. These snacks can provide a quick source of energy without causing discomfort during exercise.

By paying attention to the timing and composition of your pre-workout meals, you can optimize energy levels, improve endurance, and enhance overall exercise performance. Experiment with different options, listen to your body, and make adjustments as needed to find the pre-workout nutrition routine that works best for you.

In the upcoming chapters, we will further explore pre-workout nutrition strategies, including specific meal and snack ideas, nutrient timing, and supplementation options that can help elevate your performance during exercise.

C. Hydration and Electrolyte Balance for Peak Performance

Proper hydration and electrolyte balance are essential components of pre-performance nutrition for peak physical performance. Hydration plays a vital role in maintaining body temperature, lubricating joints, transporting nutrients, and eliminating waste products. Electrolytes, such as sodium, potassium, and magnesium, are crucial for maintaining fluid balance and supporting optimal muscle function. Consider the following guidelines to ensure proper hydration and electrolyte balance before workouts or competitions:

Hydration:

Adequate hydration should begin well before your workout or competition to ensure optimal fluid levels. Start hydrating at least a few hours before the event to allow enough time for absorption and to prevent dehydration.

- Drink water regularly throughout the day leading up to your exercise session. Aim to consume around

500-750 milliliters (16-24 ounces) of water 2-3 hours before your workout.

- Monitor your urine color: Clear or light yellow urine is a good indicator of proper hydration, while dark yellow urine may suggest dehydration.

Electrolytes:

Electrolytes are minerals that help maintain fluid balance and support various bodily functions. During intense exercise, electrolyte loss through sweat increases, which can affect performance and lead to muscle cramps or fatigue.

To ensure adequate electrolyte balance, consider the following options:

- Sports Drinks: Choose electrolyte-rich sports drinks that contain sodium, potassium, and magnesium. These drinks can help replenish electrolytes lost through sweat during prolonged or intense exercise.

- Natural Sources: Include electrolyte-rich foods in your pre-performance meal or snack. Fruits such as bananas, oranges, and watermelon contain potassium and magnesium. Salty snacks like pretzels or electrolyte-infused beverages can provide sodium.

Personalized Hydration Plan:

Hydration needs can vary based on factors such as body weight, sweat rate, and exercise intensity. It's important to develop a personalized hydration plan that suits your individual needs. Consider the following strategies:

- Determine your sweat rate: Weigh yourself before and after a workout to estimate how much fluid you lose through sweat. For every pound lost, aim to drink around 16-24 ounces of fluid to replace it.

- Hydration during Exercise: Depending on the duration and intensity of your workout, sip on water or a sports drink during exercise to maintain fluid balance.

Caffeine and Alcohol:

Limit your intake of caffeine and alcohol, as these substances can have diuretic effects and contribute to dehydration. If you consume beverages containing caffeine or alcohol, ensure you drink additional water to compensate for their dehydrating effects.

Weather Considerations:

Adjust your hydration plan based on environmental conditions. Hot and humid weather can increase fluid loss through sweat, requiring more attention to hydration. Consider increasing fluid intake during exercise in these conditions.

Remember that hydration needs are individual, so it's important to experiment and find what works best for you. Monitor your hydration status, listen to your body's cues, and make adjustments accordingly.

In the forthcoming chapters, we will delve deeper into post-performance hydration strategies, discuss rehydration techniques, and explore the role of electrolytes in recovery to further optimize your performance and overall well-being.

CHAPTER VI
Post-Performance Nutrition Strategies

A. Recovery Nutrition and the Importance of Nutrient Timing

After intense workouts or competitions, your body requires proper nutrition to recover, repair damaged tissues, replenish energy stores, and optimize performance for future activities. Post-performance nutrition plays a crucial role in facilitating these processes and ensuring optimal recovery. The timing and composition of your post-performance meal or snack are essential factors to consider. Here's why nutrient timing is important and how you can optimize your recovery nutrition:

The Anabolic Window:

The post-performance period is often referred to as the "anabolic window," a timeframe when your body is primed to absorb and utilize nutrients most efficiently. Consuming a well-balanced meal or snack within this window helps maximize the benefits of recovery nutrition.

Carbohydrates for Glycogen Replenishment:

During intense exercise, your body utilizes glycogen, the stored form of carbohydrates, as a primary fuel source. Consuming carbohydrates after your workout helps replenish glycogen stores and supports muscle recovery. Opt for complex carbohydrates like whole grains, fruits, and starchy vegetables. Aim for a carbohydrate intake of approximately 0.5-0.7 grams per pound of body weight within the first hour post-performance.

Protein for Muscle Repair and Synthesis:

Protein is crucial for muscle repair and synthesis, helping to rebuild and strengthen muscles after exercise-induced damage. Including a source of high-quality protein in your post-performance meal or snack is essential. Opt for lean protein sources such as chicken, fish, eggs, tofu, or dairy products. Aim for a protein intake of approximately 20-30 grams within the first hour post-performance.

Nutrient Timing:

Consuming a combination of carbohydrates and protein within the first hour post-performance is particularly beneficial due to enhanced nutrient uptake and muscle sensitivity to insulin during this timeframe. This combination stimulates muscle protein synthesis, leading to improved recovery and adaptation.

Fluid and Electrolyte Replenishment:

Rehydration is crucial after exercise to replenish fluid and electrolyte losses through sweat. Consume water or a sports drink that contains electrolytes to restore optimal hydration and aid in the recovery process.

Antioxidants and Anti-Inflammatory Foods:

Include foods rich in antioxidants and anti-inflammatory properties to counteract exercise-induced oxidative stress and inflammation. Colorful fruits and vegetables, nuts, seeds, and fatty fish like salmon are excellent choices. These foods provide essential nutrients that support recovery and overall health.

Meal or Snack Options:

Choose easily digestible and convenient meal or snack options to facilitate post-performance nutrition. Consider options such as a protein shake with fruits, a turkey and avocado wrap, Greek yogurt with berries, or a chicken and vegetable stir-fry with brown rice. Tailor your choices to your preferences and dietary needs.

Remember, nutrient timing is not limited to immediately after exercise. It is important to continue nourishing your body with balanced meals and snacks throughout the day to support ongoing recovery and adaptation.

In the upcoming chapters, we will explore more in-depth strategies for post-performance nutrition, including meal planning, supplementation, and practical tips for optimizing recovery to help you achieve peak performance in your athletic endeavors.

B. Replenishing Glycogen Stores and Promoting Muscle Repair

After a strenuous workout or competition, it is crucial to replenish glycogen stores and promote muscle repair to optimize recovery and prepare your body for future performances. Proper nutrition during the post-performance period plays a significant role in achieving these goals. Consider the following strategies to replenish glycogen stores and promote muscle repair:

Carbohydrate Intake:

Carbohydrates are the primary source of fuel for your muscles, and replenishing glycogen stores is essential for restoring energy levels. Aim to consume high-quality carbohydrates in your post-performance meal or snack.

- Include complex carbohydrates such as whole grains, quinoa, sweet potatoes, and brown rice. These foods provide a steady release of glucose, aiding in glycogen replenishment.

- Aim for a carbohydrate intake of approximately 1-1.5 grams per kilogram of body weight within the first hour after exercise. For example, if you weigh 70 kilograms, aim for 70-105 grams of carbohydrates.

Protein Consumption:

Protein is essential for muscle repair and growth. It provides the necessary building blocks (amino acids) to repair damaged muscle tissue and stimulate muscle protein synthesis. Including an adequate amount of protein in your post-performance nutrition is crucial.

- Opt for high-quality protein sources such as lean meats, poultry, fish, eggs, dairy products, legumes, and tofu.

- Aim for a protein intake of approximately 20-30 grams within the first hour after exercise. This amount has been shown to maximize muscle protein synthesis.

Combination of Carbohydrates and Protein:

Consuming a combination of carbohydrates and protein post-performance has shown enhanced glycogen resynthesis and muscle protein synthesis compared to consuming either nutrient alone.

- Consider options such as a turkey sandwich on whole grain bread, Greek yogurt with fruits, or a protein smoothie with added carbohydrates.

- Aim for a ratio of approximately 3:1 or 4:1 of carbohydrates to protein to optimize glycogen replenishment and muscle repair.

Timing of Nutrient Intake:

The timing of your post-performance nutrition is crucial to take advantage of the body's enhanced nutrient uptake. Ideally, consume your meal or snack within 30 minutes to 2 hours after exercise to maximize glycogen resynthesis and muscle recovery.

- If you are unable to have a complete meal, opt for a post-workout snack that provides carbohydrates and protein in the recommended amounts.

- Remember that nutrient timing is important, but overall daily nutrient intake is equally crucial. Ensure you meet your daily energy and nutrient needs through balanced meals and snacks.

Hydration and Electrolyte Balance:

Proper hydration and electrolyte balance are essential for optimal recovery. Rehydrate with water or a sports drink containing electrolytes to replace fluids lost through sweat.

Antioxidant-Rich Foods:

Include foods rich in antioxidants, such as fruits, vegetables, nuts, and seeds. These foods help reduce exercise-induced oxidative stress and inflammation, supporting muscle recovery and overall health.

By focusing on replenishing glycogen stores and promoting muscle repair through a balanced combination of carbohydrates, protein, and hydration, you can optimize recovery and set the stage for future peak performances. Experiment with different post-performance meal or snack options to find what works best for you, considering your dietary preferences and individual needs.

In the upcoming chapters, we will delve further into advanced recovery strategies, supplementation options, and practical tips to maximize your post-performance nutrition and accelerate your progress toward peak performance.

C. Adequate Hydration and Electrolyte Replacement Post-Performance

Proper hydration and electrolyte replacement are essential components of post-performance nutrition to support optimal recovery, rehydration, and overall well-being. After intense workouts or competitions, your body may be dehydrated and have depleted electrolyte levels. Here are some guidelines to ensure adequate hydration and electrolyte replacement during the post-performance period:

Rehydration Importance:

Replenishing fluids lost through sweat is crucial for rehydration and restoring optimal hydration levels. During exercise, you lose water and electrolytes, such as sodium and potassium, which need to be replenished.

Water Intake:

Water should be your primary source of rehydration. Drink water consistently after exercise to replace fluid losses. Aim to consume approximately 16-24 ounces (500-750 milliliters) of water for every pound (0.45 kilograms) of body weight lost during exercise.

Electrolyte Replacement:

Electrolytes, including sodium, potassium, magnesium, and chloride, play essential roles in maintaining fluid balance and supporting various bodily functions. Replenishing these electrolytes is crucial to restore optimal levels and promote proper muscle function.

- Sports Drinks: Consider consuming electrolyte-rich sports drinks to replenish electrolytes lost during exercise. These beverages typically contain sodium, potassium, and sometimes magnesium, aiding in electrolyte replacement. Look for drinks with balanced electrolyte compositions and avoid those with excessive added sugars.

- Electrolyte Supplements: In certain situations, such as prolonged or intense exercise, or if you are a heavy sweater, electrolyte supplements may be beneficial. Consult with a healthcare professional or sports nutritionist for personalized recommendations.

Timing of Hydration and Electrolyte Replacement:

It is important to begin rehydration and electrolyte replacement as soon as possible after exercise to optimize recovery. Aim to start rehydrating within the first hour post-performance and continue to drink fluids throughout the day.

Monitor Hydration Status:

Monitoring your hydration status can help ensure adequate rehydration. Pay attention to your urine color. Clear or light yellow urine indicates proper hydration, while dark yellow urine suggests dehydration.

Additionally, monitoring body weight changes before and after exercise can provide insights into your fluid losses.

Personalized Hydration Plan:

Individual hydration needs can vary based on factors such as body weight, exercise intensity, environmental conditions, and personal sweat rate. Develop a personalized hydration plan that suits your specific needs. Consider factors like the duration and intensity of your workouts, climate conditions, and your own hydration preferences.

Beyond Water and Sports Drinks:

Remember that hydration can come from sources other than just water and sports drinks. Fresh fruits and vegetables with high water content, such as watermelon, cucumber, and oranges, can also contribute to rehydration. Soups, smoothies, and herbal teas are additional options to increase fluid intake.

Maintaining adequate hydration and electrolyte balance is essential for optimal recovery, performance, and overall health. By incorporating these strategies into your post-performance nutrition routine, you can support efficient rehydration and electrolyte replacement, promoting proper muscle function and preparing your body for future endeavors.

In the upcoming chapters, we will explore advanced hydration strategies, discuss the impact of hydration on performance, and provide practical tips to help you optimize your post-performance nutrition and recovery process.

CHAPTER VII
Optimizing Nutrition for Specific Sports

A. Nutritional Considerations for Endurance Athletes

Endurance athletes, such as long-distance runners, cyclists, swimmers, and triathletes, have unique nutritional needs due to the prolonged and intense nature of their activities. To perform at their best and support their training and recovery, endurance athletes should pay close attention to their nutrition. Here are some key nutritional considerations for endurance athletes:

Energy Requirements:

Endurance athletes have higher energy needs compared to sedentary individuals or those involved in less demanding activities. The longer duration and higher intensity of endurance training require a sufficient intake of calories to fuel performance and promote optimal recovery.

- Calculate your daily energy needs based on your basal metabolic rate (BMR), activity level, and training volume. Work with a sports dietitian or nutritionist to determine the appropriate calorie intake for your specific needs.

Carbohydrate Loading:

Carbohydrates are the primary fuel source for endurance activities. Carbohydrate loading, also known as glycogen loading, involves increasing carbohydrate intake before a prolonged event to maximize glycogen stores in the muscles and liver.

- Gradually increase your carbohydrate intake in the days leading up to an important endurance event. Focus on consuming complex carbohydrates from sources such as whole grains, fruits, vegetables, and legumes.

- Aim to consume around 8-10 grams of carbohydrates per kilogram of body weight during the loading phase.

Hydration:

Proper hydration is crucial for endurance athletes to maintain performance, prevent dehydration, and support recovery. Fluid needs vary depending on factors such as body weight, training intensity, environmental conditions, and individual sweat rates.

- Develop a personalized hydration plan that includes regular fluid intake during training sessions and events. Monitor your fluid losses by weighing yourself before and after exercise to determine your sweat rate.

- Consume fluids before, during, and after training sessions to maintain hydration. Water, sports drinks, and electrolyte solutions can help replenish fluids and electrolytes lost through sweat.

Fueling During Endurance Activities:

During prolonged endurance activities, it is important to consume carbohydrates to maintain energy levels and delay fatigue. The type, amount, and timing of carbohydrate consumption during exercise can impact performance.

- Aim to consume 30-60 grams of carbohydrates per hour of exercise. Experiment with different forms of easily digestible carbohydrates, such as energy gels, sports drinks, or carbohydrate-rich snacks.

- Practice fueling strategies during training to determine what works best for your body and digestive system.

Recovery Nutrition:

Optimizing post-exercise nutrition is crucial for endurance athletes to replenish glycogen stores, support muscle repair, and promote recovery.

- Consume a carbohydrate-rich snack or meal within 30 minutes to an hour after training or competing to kick-start the recovery process.

- Include a source of high-quality protein to aid in muscle repair and synthesis.

- Aim for a ratio of 3:1 or 4:1 carbohydrates to protein in your post-exercise meal or snack.

Micronutrient Considerations:

Endurance athletes should ensure an adequate intake of vitamins, minerals, and antioxidants to support overall health, immune function, and performance.

- Consume a variety of nutrient-dense foods, including fruits, vegetables, whole grains, lean proteins, and healthy fats.

- Consider supplementation if your diet falls short in meeting your micronutrient needs. Consult with a healthcare professional or sports dietitian for personalized recommendations.

Endurance athletes face unique challenges when it comes to nutrition, given the demands of their training and competitions. By understanding and implementing these nutritional considerations, you can optimize your energy levels, enhance performance, and support your overall health as an endurance athlete.

In the following chapters, we will explore specific nutritional strategies for athletes in different sports, providing tailored advice to help you achieve peak performance in your chosen endurance activity.

B. Nutrition Strategies for Strength and Power-Based Sports

Strength and power-based sports, such as weightlifting, powerlifting, sprinting, and gymnastics, require athletes to generate high levels of force and power in short bursts. To excel in these sports and support muscle strength, power, and recovery, specific nutrition strategies are crucial. Here are key nutritional considerations for athletes participating in strength and power-based sports:

Energy Requirements:

Athletes involved in strength and power-based sports have higher energy requirements to support intense training sessions and muscle growth. It is important to consume enough calories to meet the energy demands of your sport and promote optimal performance.

- Calculate your daily energy needs based on your basal metabolic rate (BMR), activity level, and training volume. Work with a sports dietitian or nutritionist to determine the appropriate calorie intake for your specific needs.

Protein Intake:

Protein plays a vital role in muscle repair, recovery, and growth. Athletes in strength and power-based sports need higher protein intake to support muscle protein synthesis.

- Aim for a protein intake of approximately 1.6-2.2 grams per kilogram of body weight per day. Distribute protein intake evenly throughout the day, including sources such as lean meats, poultry, fish, eggs, dairy products, legumes, and protein supplements if needed.

Carbohydrates for Energy:

While strength and power-based sports do not rely as heavily on carbohydrates as endurance sports do, carbohydrates are still important for energy production and optimal performance.

- Consume carbohydrates from sources such as whole grains, fruits, vegetables, and legumes to provide energy for training sessions and aid in glycogen replenishment.

- Prioritize carbohydrate intake before and after workouts to fuel performance and promote recovery.

Timing of Nutrition:

The timing of meals and snacks is crucial for maximizing performance and promoting muscle recovery in strength and power-based sports.

- Consume a balanced meal or snack containing carbohydrates and protein within 1-2 hours before training sessions or competitions to provide fuel for the workout.

- After exercise, prioritize post-workout nutrition within 30 minutes to an hour to optimize muscle recovery and replenish glycogen stores.

Hydration:

Proper hydration is essential for athletes in strength and power-based sports to maintain performance, support muscle function, and prevent fatigue.

- Drink fluids regularly throughout the day, and pay attention to your body's hydration cues during training sessions.

- Consume water or sports drinks containing electrolytes to replenish fluids and electrolytes lost through sweat.

Micronutrients and Supplements:

Ensure adequate intake of vitamins, minerals, and antioxidants to support overall health and performance. While a balanced diet can provide most necessary nutrients, certain supplements may be beneficial for athletes in strength and power-based sports.

- Consult with a sports dietitian or healthcare professional to assess your individual needs and determine if supplementation is necessary.

Body Composition Considerations:

Athletes in strength and power-based sports often focus on optimizing body composition, such as increasing muscle mass or reducing body fat. Nutrition plays a critical role in achieving these goals.

- Work with a sports dietitian or nutritionist to develop a personalized nutrition plan that aligns with your body composition goals while supporting performance and overall health.

By implementing these nutrition strategies tailored to strength and power-based sports, you can enhance your performance, support muscle strength and power, and promote optimal recovery. Remember that individual needs may vary, so it is important to consult with a qualified professional to develop a nutrition plan specific to your sport and personal goals.

In the subsequent chapters, we will delve into specific nutritional strategies for athletes in different sports, providing targeted advice to help you optimize your nutrition and excel in your chosen strength and power-based sport.

C. Tailoring Nutrition for Team Sports and Intermittent Activities

Team sports and intermittent activities, such as soccer, basketball, rugby, and tennis, require a combination of endurance, power, agility, and quick recovery between intense bouts of activity. To perform at your best and support your body's demands in these sports, it is important to tailor your nutrition accordingly. Here are key nutritional considerations for athletes participating in team sports and intermittent activities:

Energy Requirements:

Athletes engaged in team sports and intermittent activities need to fuel their bodies for both endurance and bursts of high-intensity efforts. Adequate energy intake is crucial to support performance, optimize recovery, and meet the demands of training and competition.

- Calculate your daily energy needs based on your basal metabolic rate (BMR), activity level, and training volume. Work with a sports dietitian or nutritionist to determine the appropriate calorie intake for your specific needs.

Carbohydrates for Endurance and Quick Energy:

Carbohydrates play a vital role in fueling both the endurance component and the quick bursts of energy required in team sports and intermittent activities.

- Emphasize complex carbohydrates, such as whole grains, fruits, vegetables, and legumes, to provide sustained energy throughout the game or training session.

- Include some easily digestible carbohydrates, such as sports drinks, energy gels, or fruit, for quick energy during intense periods of activity.

Protein for Muscle Repair and Recovery:

Protein is essential for muscle repair and recovery, supporting the demands of team sports and intermittent activities.

- Aim for a protein intake of approximately 1.2-2.0 grams per kilogram of body weight per day to support muscle protein synthesis and repair.

- Include high-quality protein sources, such as lean meats, poultry, fish, eggs, dairy products, legumes, and plant-based proteins, in your meals and snacks.

Hydration:

Proper hydration is critical for athletes participating in team sports and intermittent activities to maintain performance, prevent dehydration, and support recovery.

- Drink fluids before, during, and after training sessions or games to maintain hydration.

- Monitor your urine color and aim for pale yellow urine as an indicator of adequate hydration.

- Consider using sports drinks that contain electrolytes during intense or prolonged activities to replenish fluids and electrolytes lost through sweat.

Timing of Nutrition:

The timing of meals and snacks is important for optimizing performance, energy levels, and recovery in team sports and intermittent activities.

- Consume a balanced meal containing carbohydrates, protein, and healthy fats 2-3 hours before training sessions or games to provide sustained energy.

- During longer matches or tournaments, consume small, easily digestible snacks or sports drinks to maintain energy levels and support endurance.

Recovery Nutrition:

Optimizing post-activity nutrition is crucial for promoting muscle recovery and glycogen replenishment in team sports and intermittent activities.

- Consume a combination of carbohydrates and protein within 30 minutes to an hour after training or competition to kick-start the recovery process.

- Include nutrient-dense foods, such as lean proteins, whole grains, fruits, vegetables, and healthy fats, in your post-activity meals and snacks.

Micronutrient Considerations:

Ensure adequate intake of vitamins, minerals, and antioxidants to support overall health, immune function, and performance.

- Consume a varied diet that includes a range of fruits, vegetables, whole grains, lean proteins, and healthy fats to obtain a broad spectrum of nutrients.

- Consider working with a sports dietitian or healthcare professional to address specific micronutrient needs based on your sport and individual requirements.

By tailoring your nutrition to the demands of team sports and intermittent activities, you can optimize your performance, support recovery, and maintain overall health. Remember that individual needs may vary, so it is important to consult with a qualified professional to develop a nutrition plan specific to your sport and personal goals.

In the upcoming chapters, we will explore specific nutritional strategies for athletes in different sports, providing targeted advice to help you excel in your chosen team sport or intermittent activity.

CHAPTER VIII
Supplementation for Performance Enhancement

A. Understanding the Role of Supplements in Performance Nutrition

Supplements are commonly used by athletes to enhance performance, improve recovery, and optimize nutritional status. While a well-rounded and balanced diet should provide most of the necessary nutrients, certain supplements may be beneficial in specific situations. It is essential to have a clear understanding of the role of supplements in performance nutrition. Here are key points to consider:

Supplementation as a Supplement, Not a Replacement:

Supplements should be viewed as additions to a healthy and balanced diet, not substitutes for whole foods. They are intended to fill nutrient gaps or address specific needs that cannot be adequately met through dietary sources alone.

Nutritional Deficiencies and Specific Needs:

Supplements can be helpful when addressing nutritional deficiencies or specific nutrient needs. For example, athletes with limited sun exposure might benefit from vitamin D supplementation, or those with inadequate dietary intake of omega-3 fatty acids might consider fish oil supplements.

Ergogenic Aids:

Some supplements are marketed as ergogenic aids, claiming to enhance performance, strength, or endurance. However, the efficacy and safety of many of these products are still subject to debate and further scientific research. It is important to approach such claims with skepticism and seek evidence-based information.

Individual Variations:

Individual responses to supplements can vary significantly. What works for one athlete may not have the same effect on another. Factors such as genetics, diet, training regimen, and overall health can influence the effectiveness and suitability of supplements for each individual.

Quality and Safety:

When considering supplements, it is crucial to prioritize quality and safety. Choose reputable brands that undergo third-party testing to ensure product purity and accurate labeling. Additionally, consult with a healthcare professional or sports dietitian to assess the safety and potential interactions of any supplements with medications or existing health conditions.

Legal and Banned Substances:

Athletes should be aware of the regulations and guidelines set by their respective sports organizations regarding the use of supplements and banned substances. Some supplements may contain ingredients that are prohibited in competitive sports. It is important to carefully read labels and consult with a knowledgeable professional to avoid inadvertent violations.

Personalized Approach:

The decision to use supplements should be based on individual needs, goals, and informed choices. A personalized approach, taking into account factors such as training load, dietary patterns, and specific requirements, can help determine whether supplementation is appropriate and beneficial for an athlete.

Sports-Specific Considerations:

Certain sports may have unique nutritional requirements, which may influence the use of supplements. For example, endurance athletes might benefit from carbohydrate-electrolyte drinks or gels during prolonged exercise, while strength athletes might consider creatine supplementation to support power and strength gains.

Remember, while supplements may have a place in performance nutrition, they should never replace a well-balanced diet and a foundation of healthy eating habits. Individualized advice from a sports dietitian or healthcare professional is invaluable in making informed decisions about supplement use, ensuring safety, and optimizing performance.

In the subsequent chapters, we will explore specific supplements commonly used in performance nutrition, discussing their potential benefits, risks, and evidence-based recommendations.

B. Exploring Commonly Used Supplements and Their Effectiveness

Supplements are widely used by athletes seeking an extra edge in their performance and recovery. While scientific evidence for many supplements is still evolving, some have been extensively studied for their potential benefits. Here, we explore commonly used supplements and their effectiveness:

Creatine:

Creatine is one of the most popular and well-researched supplements for improving strength, power, and muscle mass. It helps replenish adenosine triphosphate (ATP), the primary energy source for muscle contractions.

- Numerous studies have shown that creatine supplementation can enhance high-intensity exercise performance, particularly in activities that involve short bursts of maximal effort, such as weightlifting and sprinting.

Caffeine:

Caffeine is a stimulant that can increase alertness, reduce fatigue, and improve endurance performance. It stimulates the central nervous system and enhances the utilization of fat as a fuel source.

- Research suggests that caffeine can enhance endurance performance, especially in activities lasting longer than 30 minutes. It may also improve focus and concentration during training or competition.

Beta-Alanine:

Beta-alanine is an amino acid that increases muscle carnosine levels. Carnosine acts as a buffer, helping to reduce muscle acidity and delay fatigue during high-intensity exercise.

- Studies have demonstrated that beta-alanine supplementation can improve exercise capacity and performance in activities lasting 1-4 minutes, such as repeated sprints or high-intensity interval training (HIIT).

Branched-Chain Amino Acids (BCAAs):

BCAAs, including leucine, isoleucine, and valine, are essential amino acids that play a role in muscle protein synthesis and reduce exercise-induced muscle damage.

- While BCAAs are commonly used, their effectiveness in improving performance or reducing muscle soreness is still debated. Current evidence suggests that their benefits may be more prominent in situations of prolonged endurance exercise or during periods of energy restriction.

Nitric Oxide Boosters:

Nitric oxide (NO) boosters, such as arginine and citrulline, are thought to enhance blood flow, increase oxygen and nutrient delivery to muscles, and improve endurance performance.

- The evidence on the effectiveness of NO boosters is mixed. Some studies have reported improvements in exercise performance and cardiovascular function, while others have not shown significant benefits. More research is needed to establish their efficacy.

Vitamin D:

Vitamin D plays a crucial role in bone health, immune function, and muscle function. It also regulates calcium absorption and is involved in various physiological processes.

- Athletes with vitamin D deficiency may benefit from supplementation to maintain adequate levels. However, the benefits of vitamin D supplementation on performance outcomes are not yet well-established.

It is important to note that individual responses to supplements can vary, and the effectiveness of supplements may depend on factors such as training status, diet, and specific sport requirements. Moreover, supplements should always be used in conjunction with a well-balanced diet and under the guidance of a healthcare professional or sports dietitian.

In the subsequent chapters, we will delve deeper into specific supplements, discussing dosage recommendations, potential side effects, and the current scientific evidence supporting their use. Remember to consult with a qualified professional to determine the most appropriate supplements for your individual needs and goals.

B. Exploring Commonly Used Supplements and Their Effectiveness

When it comes to performance enhancement, athletes often turn to supplements to boost their results. While some supplements have demonstrated positive effects in certain areas, it is crucial to understand their effectiveness and potential risks. Let's explore some commonly used supplements and their impact on performance:

Creatine:

Creatine is a naturally occurring compound found in meat and fish. It has been extensively studied for its ability to enhance high-intensity, short-duration activities.

- Research consistently shows that creatine supplementation can increase strength, power, and muscle mass. It improves ATP resynthesis, allowing athletes to perform at higher intensities for longer durations.

Caffeine:

Caffeine is a stimulant that is widely consumed for its ability to increase alertness and reduce fatigue. It acts on the central nervous system and has been shown to enhance performance in endurance and team sports.

- Caffeine can improve endurance exercise performance by stimulating the release of fatty acids, which serve as an additional fuel source. It may also reduce the perception of effort and increase focus and concentration.

Beta-Alanine:

Beta-alanine is an amino acid that combines with histidine to form carnosine, which helps buffer acidity in the muscles. This buffering effect delays muscle fatigue during high-intensity exercise.

- Research indicates that beta-alanine supplementation can improve performance in activities lasting 1-4 minutes, such as repeated sprints or interval training. It is particularly beneficial for exercises that rely on anaerobic metabolism.

Branched-Chain Amino Acids (BCAAs):

BCAAs consist of three essential amino acids: leucine, isoleucine, and valine. They are popular among athletes for their potential role in muscle recovery and reducing muscle soreness.

- While BCAAs are commonly consumed, the scientific evidence supporting their effectiveness is limited. They may have some benefits during prolonged endurance exercise or in situations of energy restriction, but their overall impact on performance remains uncertain.

Nitric Oxide Boosters:

Nitric oxide boosters, such as arginine and citrulline, are believed to enhance blood flow, improve oxygen delivery, and promote nutrient uptake in muscles.

- While these supplements are marketed for improving performance, the scientific evidence is inconclusive. Some studies suggest a potential benefit in endurance performance, while others do not show significant effects. Further research is needed to draw definitive conclusions.

Vitamin D:

Vitamin D plays a vital role in bone health, immune function, and muscle strength. Athletes with low vitamin D levels may consider supplementation to optimize performance and overall health.

- Vitamin D supplementation is beneficial for individuals with deficiency, as it supports calcium absorption and muscle function. However, the impact of vitamin D on performance outcomes is still being investigated.

It's important to note that individual responses to supplements can vary, and their effectiveness may depend on factors such as training status, diet, and specific sport requirements. Additionally, supplements should be used with caution and under the guidance of a healthcare professional or sports nutritionist.

In the following chapters, we will explore specific supplements in more detail, discussing dosages, potential side effects, and the current scientific evidence supporting their use. Remember to prioritize a well-balanced diet and seek professional advice before incorporating supplements into your routine.

C. Risks, Benefits, and Guidelines for Responsible Supplementation

While supplements can offer potential benefits for performance enhancement, it is crucial to approach supplementation responsibly. Understanding the risks and benefits associated with supplements and following appropriate guidelines is essential. Here, we explore the risks, benefits, and guidelines for responsible supplementation:

Risks of Supplementation:

a. Contamination: Some supplements may contain impurities or substances not listed on the label, posing potential health risks. Choosing reputable brands that undergo third-party testing can minimize this risk.

b. Adverse Effects: Certain supplements can cause side effects, ranging from mild discomfort to serious health complications. It is important to be aware of potential side effects and consult a healthcare professional before starting any new supplement.

c. Drug Interactions: Supplements may interact with medications, altering their effectiveness or causing adverse reactions. Always disclose all supplements you are taking to your healthcare provider to avoid potential interactions.

Benefits of Responsible Supplementation:

a. Addressing Nutrient Deficiencies: Supplements can help fill nutritional gaps when certain nutrients are lacking in the diet, supporting overall health and performance.

b. Meeting Increased Demands: Intense training and competition may increase nutrient requirements beyond what can be met through diet alone. Supplements can help ensure athletes meet these increased demands.

c. Convenience and Practicality: In some cases, supplements can provide a convenient and practical way to meet specific nutritional needs, especially when whole food options may be limited.

Guidelines for Responsible Supplementation:

a. Individualized Approach: Each athlete has unique nutritional needs. Tailor supplement use based on personal goals, sport, training load, and health status. Consulting with a qualified professional can help develop an individualized plan.

b. Quality and Safety: Choose supplements from reputable manufacturers that follow Good Manufacturing Practices (GMP) and undergo third-party testing. Look for certifications, such as NSF Certified for Sport or Informed-Sport, to ensure quality and purity.

c. Evidence-Based Decisions: Seek out supplements with a strong scientific evidence base supporting their effectiveness. Be cautious of exaggerated claims or products lacking substantial research.

d. Transparent Labeling: Read supplement labels carefully to understand ingredients, dosage recommendations, and potential allergens. Look for supplements that provide transparent and accurate information.

e. Regular Monitoring: Regularly assess the need for supplementation as nutritional requirements may change over time. Monitor your response to supplements and make adjustments as needed.

f. Periodic Review: Re-evaluate the necessity and effectiveness of supplements periodically. As new research emerges, recommendations may change, so staying informed is crucial.

g. Education and Professional Guidance: Stay informed about supplements through reputable sources, such as sports dietitians, certified sports nutritionists, or reputable scientific publications. Seek professional guidance for personalized advice.

Remember, supplements should complement a well-balanced diet, not replace it. Prioritize whole, nutrient-dense foods as the foundation of your nutrition plan. Always consult with a healthcare professional or sports nutritionist before initiating any new supplement regimen.

In the subsequent chapters, we will delve deeper into specific supplements, discussing their uses, potential risks, dosage recommendations, and evidence-based guidelines to support responsible supplementation.

CHAPTER IX
Overcoming Nutritional Challenges

A. Dealing with Dietary Restrictions and Allergies

Nutrition plays a critical role in fueling your body for peak performance, but it can be challenging to navigate dietary restrictions and allergies while optimizing your nutrition. Whether you have specific dietary needs due to medical conditions, allergies, or personal beliefs, there are strategies to overcome these challenges. Here, we explore how to deal with dietary restrictions and allergies:

Identify and Understand Your Restrictions:

a. Allergies: If you have food allergies, it is vital to identify the allergens and be vigilant about avoiding them. Common allergens include peanuts, tree nuts, shellfish, dairy, soy, wheat, and eggs. Read food labels carefully, inform restaurant staff about your allergies, and consider carrying allergy medication with you.

b. Medical Conditions: Certain medical conditions, such as celiac disease, lactose intolerance, or diabetes, may require specific dietary modifications. Work with a registered dietitian or healthcare professional to develop a personalized meal plan that meets your nutritional needs while managing your condition.

c. Personal Beliefs: Some individuals choose to follow specific dietary practices, such as vegetarianism, veganism, or religious dietary restrictions. Understanding the principles of these practices and finding alternative food sources to meet nutrient requirements is essential.

Seek Professional Guidance:

a. Registered Dietitian: Consulting with a registered dietitian who specializes in sports nutrition or specific dietary needs can provide invaluable guidance. They can help create a personalized meal plan, ensure nutrient adequacy, and offer practical strategies for managing restrictions.

Food Substitutions and Alternatives:

a. Allergies: Identify suitable substitutes for allergenic foods. For example, if you are allergic to dairy, explore plant-based alternatives like almond milk, coconut milk, or soy milk. Experiment with alternative flours, such as almond flour or quinoa flour, if you have a gluten allergy.

b. Medical Conditions: Work with a dietitian to find suitable alternatives that meet your nutritional requirements while accommodating your medical condition. For example, if you have celiac disease, choose gluten-free grains like quinoa, rice, or amaranth.

Meal Planning and Preparation:

a. Plan Ahead: Take time to plan your meals and snacks in advance, ensuring they align with your dietary restrictions. This will help you stay on track and avoid last-minute challenges.

b. Cooking at Home: Preparing meals at home gives you control over the ingredients and allows you to accommodate your dietary needs more easily. Experiment with new recipes and explore diverse flavors to make mealtime enjoyable.

Communication and Advocacy:

a. Restaurants and Social Gatherings: When dining out, communicate your dietary restrictions or allergies to the restaurant staff to ensure they can accommodate your needs. If attending social gatherings, inform the host about your restrictions, and offer to bring a dish that aligns with your dietary needs.

b. Educate Others: Help others understand your dietary restrictions and allergies by providing information and resources. This will foster understanding and support from friends, family, and teammates.

Remember, maintaining optimal nutrition is possible even with dietary restrictions or allergies. By staying informed, seeking professional guidance, and being proactive in your meal planning, you can overcome these challenges and fuel your body for peak performance.

In the following chapters, we will address other common nutritional challenges and provide strategies to overcome them, enabling you to achieve your performance goals while staying within the bounds of your dietary needs.

B. Strategies for Maintaining Nutrition While Traveling or Dining Out

Maintaining optimal nutrition can be challenging when traveling or dining out, as you may encounter unfamiliar foods, limited options, or tempting indulgences. However, with careful planning and smart choices, you can navigate these situations and stay on track with your nutrition goals. Here are some strategies for maintaining nutrition while traveling or dining out:

Plan Ahead:

a. Research Restaurants: Before traveling, investigate restaurants in the area that offer healthier options or cater to specific dietary needs. Look for menus online and read reviews to make informed choices.

b. Pack Snacks: Bring nutrient-dense snacks such as nuts, seeds, protein bars, or dried fruits to have on hand during travel or when healthy options are limited.

Make Smart Menu Choices:

a. Prioritize Protein and Vegetables: Look for dishes that include lean protein sources like grilled chicken, fish, or tofu, paired with a variety of colorful vegetables. This ensures you're getting essential nutrients and helps keep you satiated.

b. Opt for Whole Grains: Choose whole grain options whenever possible, such as whole wheat bread, brown rice, or quinoa. These provide more fiber and nutrients compared to refined grains.

c. Be Mindful of Portions: Restaurant servings are often larger than what you would typically consume at home. Consider sharing a dish with a friend or ask for a half portion to avoid overeating.

Customize Your Order:

a. Ask for Modifications: Don't hesitate to request modifications to suit your dietary preferences or restrictions. Ask for sauces or dressings on the side, opt for grilled or steamed preparations, and substitute ingredients when necessary.

b. Increase Vegetable Intake: If a dish doesn't include enough vegetables, ask if you can add extra veggies or request a side of steamed vegetables to enhance the nutritional value of your meal.

Stay Hydrated:

a. Carry a Water Bottle: Stay hydrated by carrying a reusable water bottle and refilling it regularly. This will help you avoid sugary beverages and maintain optimal hydration levels.

b. Limit Alcohol Consumption: Alcoholic beverages can be high in calories and have a negative impact on performance. If you choose to drink, do so in moderation and opt for lower-calorie options like light beer or a glass of wine.

Practice Mindful Eating:

a. Slow Down: Take your time to savor each bite and enjoy the dining experience. Eating slowly allows your body to recognize fullness and helps prevent overeating.

b. Listen to Your Hunger Cues: Pay attention to your body's signals of hunger and fullness. Stop eating when you feel satisfied, even if there is food left on your plate.

Stay Active:

a. Explore Active Opportunities: When traveling, make an effort to explore the local area on foot, rent bicycles, or engage in activities that keep you physically active. This helps maintain energy expenditure and supports overall well-being.

b. Use Hotel Fitness Facilities: If your accommodation provides fitness facilities, take advantage of them to continue your regular exercise routine while on the road.

By implementing these strategies, you can maintain your nutrition goals while traveling or dining out. Remember that flexibility and moderation are key. Enjoy the experience, make conscious choices, and strive for balance to fuel your body for peak performance.

In the upcoming chapters, we will address additional nutritional challenges and provide strategies to overcome them, ensuring you have the tools and knowledge to optimize your nutrition in any situation.

C. Addressing Common Obstacles to Optimal Nutrition

While striving for optimal nutrition, various obstacles can hinder your progress and impact your ability to fuel your body for peak performance. It's important to identify and address these obstacles to ensure you stay on track with your nutrition goals. Here, we explore some common challenges and provide strategies to overcome them:

Time Constraints:

a. Meal Prep: Dedicate some time each week to meal preparation. Plan and cook meals in advance, portion them into containers, and store them in the fridge or freezer for convenient access to nutritious options throughout the week.

b. Quick and Easy Recipes: Seek out simple, time-efficient recipes that require minimal ingredients and preparation.

Look for meals that can be made in one pot or use a slow cooker for effortless cooking.

Emotional Eating:

a. Recognize Triggers: Identify the emotions or situations that trigger emotional eating. Find alternative coping mechanisms such as engaging in physical activity, practicing relaxation techniques, or seeking support from friends or a therapist.

b. Mindful Eating: Practice mindful eating by paying attention to your hunger and fullness cues. Slow down, savor each bite, and be present in the moment. This helps prevent mindless eating and promotes a healthier relationship with food.

Cravings and Temptations:

a. Find Healthy Alternatives: Identify healthier alternatives to satisfy cravings. For example, if you crave something sweet, reach for a piece of fruit or opt for a small portion of dark chocolate.

b. Practice Moderation: Allow yourself occasional treats or indulgences while being mindful of portion sizes. Enjoy the foods you love in moderation, balancing them with nutrient-dense meals and snacks.

Lack of Support:

a. Communicate Your Goals: Share your nutrition goals and aspirations with supportive friends, family, or teammates. Explain the importance of your journey and how their encouragement and understanding can help you stay on track.

b. Seek Like-Minded Communities: Join online forums, social media groups, or local organizations focused on nutrition and healthy lifestyles. Surrounding yourself with individuals who share similar goals can provide motivation, inspiration, and a sense of community.

Limited Access to Fresh Foods:

a. Prioritize Nutrient-Dense Options: Make the best choices with the available resources. Select whole, minimally processed foods that offer the most nutritional value, such as fruits, vegetables, lean proteins, and whole grains.

b. Explore Frozen and Canned Options: When fresh produce is scarce or expensive, consider frozen or canned alternatives. These options can still provide valuable nutrients and be a convenient solution.

Stress and Busy Lifestyles:

a. Practice Stress Management: Incorporate stress-management techniques such as exercise, meditation, deep breathing exercises, or engaging in hobbies. These strategies help reduce stress levels and prevent stress-induced unhealthy eating habits.

b. Simplify Meal Planning: Opt for quick and easy meal options during particularly busy periods. Choose recipes with minimal ingredients or consider meal delivery services that provide healthy, pre-prepared options.

By addressing these common obstacles to optimal nutrition, you can overcome challenges and continue on your journey toward peak performance. Remember that small steps and consistent efforts make a significant difference. Stay committed, adapt to your circumstances, and seek support when needed.

In the upcoming chapters, we will explore further nutritional challenges and provide effective strategies to conquer them, ensuring you have the knowledge and tools to overcome any obstacle that comes your way.

CHAPTER X
Long-Term Nutrition and Lifestyle Habits

A. Developing Sustainable Eating Habits for Lasting Results

Achieving optimal nutrition and peak performance is not just about short-term changes; it's about developing sustainable eating habits that can be maintained over the long term. Building a solid foundation of healthy practices ensures lasting results and promotes overall well-being. Here are some strategies to help you develop sustainable eating habits:

Set Realistic Goals:

a. Define Your Objectives: Clearly identify your nutrition goals and what you aim to achieve. Whether it's improving performance, maintaining weight, or enhancing overall health, setting realistic and specific goals provides clarity and direction.

b. Break It Down: Divide your goals into smaller, achievable steps. Focus on making gradual changes that are easier to incorporate into your lifestyle rather than overwhelming yourself with drastic modifications.

Adopt a Balanced Approach:

a. Embrace Variety: Include a wide range of foods from different food groups in your diet. This ensures you receive a diverse array of nutrients necessary for optimal performance and overall health.

b. Practice Portion Control: Be mindful of portion sizes to avoid overeating. Use visual cues, such as hand sizes or measuring cups, to gauge appropriate serving sizes.

Listen to Your Body:

a. Honor Hunger and Fullness: Pay attention to your body's signals of hunger and fullness. Eat when you're hungry and stop when you're satisfied, rather than relying on external cues or eating out of habit.

b. Practice Intuitive Eating: Tune into your body's needs and preferences. Give yourself permission to enjoy a variety of foods without guilt or restrictions, while staying attuned to how certain foods make you feel.

Plan and Prepare:

a. Meal Planning: Devote time to plan your meals and snacks for the week. This helps you make healthier choices, saves time, and reduces reliance on less nutritious options.

b. Healthy Food Choices: Stock your pantry, refrigerator, and freezer with nutritious options. Having a variety of healthy ingredients readily available makes it easier to prepare balanced meals and snacks.

Seek Support and Accountability:

a. Share Your Journey: Inform friends, family, or a supportive community about your goals. Having a support system can provide encouragement, motivation, and accountability.

b. Find an Accountability Partner: Consider partnering with someone who shares similar nutrition and performance goals. You can hold each other accountable, share successes and challenges, and provide mutual support.

Adapt and Iterate:

a. Be Flexible: Recognize that life circumstances may require adjustments to your eating habits. Adapt to changes, such as travel, holidays, or personal events, while still maintaining a focus on balanced nutrition.

b. Learn from Experiences: Reflect on your nutrition choices and outcomes. Take note of what works well for you and what needs improvement, then make necessary adjustments to fine-tune your approach.

Remember, developing sustainable eating habits is a continuous process that evolves over time. It's about finding a balance that works for you, honoring your body's needs, and enjoying a varied and nourishing diet. By implementing these strategies, you can establish a foundation of healthy habits that support your long-term nutrition goals and foster lasting results.

In the following chapters, we will delve deeper into other aspects of long-term nutrition and lifestyle habits, providing valuable insights and guidance to help you on your journey to peak performance and optimal nutrition.

B. The Role of Sleep, Stress Management, and Recovery in Performance

When it comes to optimizing nutrition and achieving peak performance, it's essential to recognize the significant role that sleep, stress management, and recovery play in overall well-being. These factors not only impact your physical and mental health but also influence your ability to perform at your best. Here's a closer look at how sleep, stress management, and recovery contribute to performance:

Sleep:

Adequate and quality sleep is crucial for optimal performance. During sleep, the body undergoes essential processes that support physical and cognitive functioning. Here are key points to consider:

a. Restoration and Repair: Sleep allows the body to repair and regenerate tissues, replenish energy stores, and promote muscle recovery. It also supports immune function and hormone regulation.

b. Cognitive Functioning: Sufficient sleep enhances cognitive abilities, including attention, concentration, memory, and decision-making. It improves focus, reaction time, and problem-solving skills, all of which are vital for performance.

c. Sleep Duration and Quality: Aim for 7-9 hours of uninterrupted sleep each night. Establish a consistent sleep schedule, create a sleep-friendly environment, and practice relaxation techniques to improve sleep quality.

Stress Management:

Effective stress management techniques are crucial for maintaining optimal performance. Chronic stress can negatively impact physical and mental health, as well as hinder performance. Consider the following:

a. Mindfulness and Relaxation: Engage in activities that promote relaxation and reduce stress, such as meditation, deep breathing exercises, yoga, or tai chi. These practices help calm the mind and promote overall well-being.

b. Time Management: Prioritize tasks, set realistic goals, and establish boundaries to avoid feeling overwhelmed. Effective time management reduces stress and allows for better focus and performance.

c. Social Support: Build a support network of friends, family, or professionals who can provide guidance, understanding, and encouragement. Sharing concerns and seeking support can help alleviate stress and foster resilience.

Recovery:

Proper recovery is vital for sustained performance and injury prevention. It involves strategies that allow the body to repair and adapt after physical activity. Consider the following:

a. Active Recovery: Engage in light exercise, such as walking, stretching, or low-intensity activities, on rest days. Active recovery promotes blood flow, reduces muscle soreness, and enhances overall recovery.

b. Nutrition for Recovery: Optimize your post-workout nutrition by consuming a combination of carbohydrates and protein within the first 30-60 minutes after exercise. This helps replenish glycogen stores and supports muscle repair.

c. Rest and Relaxation: Allow yourself adequate rest periods between training sessions to prevent overtraining and promote recovery. Prioritize quality sleep and incorporate relaxation techniques into your routine.

By prioritizing sleep, managing stress effectively, and allowing for proper recovery, you can enhance your overall well-being, maintain optimal performance, and minimize the risk of burnout or injuries.

In the final chapters of this book, we will explore additional aspects of long-term nutrition and lifestyle habits, providing insights and strategies to help you sustain your performance and achieve your goals. Remember, a holistic approach that considers sleep, stress management, and recovery is key to unlocking your full potential.

C. Integrating Nutrition into a Holistic Approach to Overall Health and Well-Being

Optimal nutrition goes beyond just fueling your body for peak performance. It is an essential component of a holistic approach to overall health and well-being. When you integrate nutrition into your lifestyle, you create a solid foundation for a healthy and balanced life. Here are some ways to integrate nutrition into a holistic approach:

Mindful Eating:

a. Awareness: Practice mindful eating by paying attention to your body's hunger and fullness cues. Slow down and savor each bite, being present in the moment and fully experiencing the flavors and textures of your food.

b. Emotional Connection: Recognize the emotional aspects of eating. Understand your relationship with food and be mindful of emotional triggers that may lead to unhealthy eating patterns. Use nutrition to nourish not only your body but also your mind and soul.

Holistic Nutrition:

a. Nutrient-Dense Foods: Focus on consuming whole, unprocessed foods that are rich in essential nutrients. Include a variety of fruits, vegetables, whole grains, lean proteins, and healthy fats in your diet. These foods provide the necessary nutrients for optimal health and well-being.

b. Functional Foods: Incorporate functional foods that offer additional health benefits. For example, turmeric has anti-inflammatory properties, and probiotics promote gut health. Explore the power of food as medicine and incorporate ingredients that support your specific health needs.

Balancing Macronutrients:

a. Carbohydrates: Choose complex carbohydrates, such as whole grains and vegetables, for sustained energy levels. Avoid excessive consumption of refined carbohydrates and sugary foods, as they can lead to energy crashes and disrupt overall balance.

b. Proteins: Include lean sources of protein, such as poultry, fish, legumes, and tofu, to support muscle repair and growth. Aim for a balance between animal and plant-based protein sources.

c. Fats: Incorporate healthy fats, such as avocados, nuts, seeds, and olive oil, in moderation. These fats provide essential fatty acids and contribute to satiety and overall well-being.

Hydration:

a. Water Intake: Stay adequately hydrated by consuming enough water throughout the day. Water supports digestion, nutrient absorption, circulation, and overall bodily functions. Carry a reusable water bottle and make hydration a priority.

b. Herbal Teas and Infusions: Explore herbal teas and infusions that provide hydration along with additional health benefits. For example, green tea is rich in antioxidants, while chamomile tea promotes relaxation.

Physical Activity:

a. Complementing Nutrition: Combine proper nutrition with regular physical activity for overall health and well-being. Physical activity enhances metabolism, supports cardiovascular health, boosts mood, and contributes to weight management.

b. Energy Balance: Adjust your nutrition to support your activity level. Fuel your body with appropriate macronutrients and timing to meet the demands of your physical activity while maintaining a healthy energy balance.

Self-Care and Stress Reduction:

a. Self-Care Practices: Prioritize self-care activities that promote relaxation and stress reduction. This can include activities such as meditation, yoga, journaling, spending time in nature, or engaging in hobbies that bring you joy.

b. Emotional Well-Being: Recognize the impact of stress on your overall health. Develop coping mechanisms to manage stress effectively, such as seeking support, practicing mindfulness, or engaging in stress-reducing activities.

By integrating nutrition into a holistic approach to overall health and well-being, you create a sustainable and nourishing lifestyle. Remember, optimal nutrition is not an isolated concept but rather an integral part of a broader framework that encompasses physical, mental, and emotional well-being. Embrace the power of nutrition to support and enhance every aspect of your life.

CHAPTER XI
Conclusion

A. Recap of Key Points and Takeaways

In this book, we have explored the vital role of optimal nutrition in fueling your body for peak performance. Let's recap the key points and takeaways from our journey:

Importance of Nutrition:

- Nutrition plays a crucial role in achieving peak performance by providing the necessary fuel and nutrients for your body to function optimally.

- It impacts not only physical performance but also mental clarity, focus, and overall well-being.

Understanding Nutrition:

- Macronutrients (carbohydrates, proteins, and fats) and micronutrients (vitamins and minerals) are essential components of a balanced diet.

- Carbohydrates provide energy, proteins support muscle repair and growth, and fats contribute to overall health and hormone regulation.

- Vitamins and minerals are crucial for various bodily functions and should be obtained through a diverse and nutrient-dense diet.

Assessing Your Nutritional Needs:

- Determining your caloric requirements is essential for meeting your energy needs and maintaining a healthy weight.

- Analyzing your individual dietary goals and activity levels helps customize your nutrition plan for optimal performance.

Designing a Balanced Meal Plan:

- A well-balanced diet includes a variety of nutrient-dense foods that provide a wide range of essential nutrients.

- Planning meals to meet macronutrient and micronutrient requirements ensures adequate nourishment for your body.

Pre-Performance Nutrition Strategies:

- Fueling your body before workouts or competitions is crucial for optimal performance.

- Consider the timing and composition of pre-workout meals to provide the right nutrients at the right time.

Post-Performance Nutrition Strategies:

- Recovery nutrition is essential for replenishing glycogen stores, promoting muscle repair, and facilitating overall recovery.

- Adequate hydration and electrolyte replacement are vital for post-performance recovery.

Optimizing Nutrition for Specific Sports:

- Different sports have unique nutritional considerations, such as endurance athletes requiring adequate fuel and hydration, and strength and power-based sports benefiting from protein-rich diets.

Supplementation for Performance Enhancement:

- Supplements can play a role in performance nutrition, but their effectiveness varies, and responsible use is essential.

- Understanding the risks, benefits, and guidelines for responsible supplementation is crucial.

Overcoming Nutritional Challenges:

- Dealing with dietary restrictions and allergies requires careful planning and finding suitable alternatives.

- Strategies for maintaining nutrition while traveling or dining out involve making informed choices and being mindful of your food choices.

Long-Term Nutrition and Lifestyle Habits:

- Integrating nutrition into a holistic approach to overall health and well-being involves mindful eating, balancing macronutrients, prioritizing sleep, managing stress, and promoting recovery.

- Developing sustainable eating habits is essential for long-lasting results.

In conclusion, achieving optimal nutrition is a journey that requires knowledge, awareness, and commitment. By understanding the fundamentals of nutrition, assessing your specific needs, and implementing strategies for pre- and post-performance nutrition, you can fuel your body for peak performance. Remember to address common obstacles, tailor nutrition to your specific sport, and consider the role of supplements responsibly. Finally, integrating nutrition into a holistic approach to overall health and well-being ensures long-term success and sustainability.

Armed with the knowledge and insights gained from this book, you are well-equipped to make informed choices and take control of your nutrition to unlock your full potential and achieve peak performance. Here's to a future of optimal nutrition and exceptional performance!

B. Encouragement to Implement Optimal Nutrition for Peak Performance

As we conclude this journey through the world of optimal nutrition for peak performance, I want to leave you with a final message of encouragement. You now possess a wealth of knowledge about the importance of nutrition, understanding macronutrients and micronutrients, assessing your nutritional needs, designing balanced meal plans, and implementing pre- and post-performance nutrition strategies. It's time to take action and implement what you have learned to fuel your body for peak performance.

Embarking on a journey of optimal nutrition requires dedication, commitment, and a willingness to make positive changes in your lifestyle. The benefits you will reap from prioritizing your nutrition are worth every effort. By fueling your body with the right nutrients at the right times, you can enhance your physical performance, mental clarity, and overall well-being.

Remember that implementing optimal nutrition is a gradual process. Start by incorporating small changes into your daily routine. Focus on making healthier food choices, experimenting with nutrient-dense recipes, and being mindful of portion sizes. With time, these habits will become second nature, leading to a sustainable and nourishing lifestyle.

Stay motivated and keep your goals in mind. Whether you are an athlete striving for peak performance, a fitness enthusiast aiming to improve your workouts, or someone simply seeking to enhance your overall health and well-being, optimal nutrition is the key to unlocking your full potential.

Surround yourself with a supportive environment. Seek the guidance of nutrition experts, connect with like-minded individuals who share your passion for healthy living, and find accountability partners who can cheer you on throughout your journey. Remember, you are not alone in this pursuit of optimal nutrition and peak performance.

Celebrate your achievements along the way, no matter how small they may seem. Recognize that every positive step you take towards implementing optimal nutrition is a step towards a healthier, more vibrant version of yourself. Embrace the process, be patient with yourself, and trust that the results will come.

Finally, always listen to your body. Each individual is unique, and what works for one person may not work for another. Pay attention to how your body responds to different foods and adjust your nutrition plan accordingly. Remember that optimal nutrition is a dynamic and ever-evolving journey, and what works for you today may need to be adjusted in the future.

Now is the time to take what you have learned and put it into practice. Believe in yourself and the power of optimal nutrition to fuel your body for peak performance. The possibilities are endless, and your potential is limitless. Embrace the journey, make the commitment, and witness the transformative power of optimal nutrition in your life.

Here's to a future filled with energy, vitality, and the pursuit of excellence through optimal nutrition. You have all the tools you need. Now, go out there and unleash your full potential!

C. Inspiring Readers to Embrace a Lifelong Commitment to Their Nutritional Well-being

As we come to the end of this journey exploring optimal nutrition for peak performance, I want to leave you with a final message of inspiration and encouragement. Throughout this book, you have gained valuable knowledge about the importance of nutrition, understanding macronutrients and micronutrients, assessing your nutritional needs, and designing balanced meal plans. Now, it's time to embark on a lifelong commitment to your nutritional well-being.

Your health and well-being are precious assets that deserve your attention and care. By embracing a lifelong commitment to optimal nutrition, you are making a powerful investment in yourself and your future.

Remember that nutrition is not a quick fix or a temporary solution—it is a fundamental pillar of your overall well-being.

Embracing a lifelong commitment to your nutritional well-being is about more than just the food you eat. It is a holistic approach that encompasses your relationship with food, your mindset, and your lifestyle choices. It is about nourishing your body, mind, and soul.

When you prioritize optimal nutrition, you give yourself the gift of vitality, energy, and resilience. You enhance your physical performance, boost your cognitive function, and improve your overall quality of life. You become better equipped to face life's challenges with strength and grace.

Embracing a lifelong commitment to optimal nutrition does not mean striving for perfection or adhering to strict rules. It means finding balance, flexibility, and self-compassion in your approach. It means making informed choices and being mindful of how the food you eat nourishes your body.

Remember that optimal nutrition is not a destination but a continuous journey. It evolves as you grow, change, and face new experiences. Be open to learning, exploring, and adapting your nutritional choices along the way. Seek out new information, experiment with different foods, and listen to your body's wisdom.

Surround yourself with a supportive community that shares your passion for health and wellness. Connect with others who inspire and uplift you on your journey. Share your knowledge, experiences, and challenges. Together, we can create a culture that values and prioritizes optimal nutrition for everyone.

Embrace the joy of food and the pleasure of nourishing your body. Explore the rich variety of flavors, textures, and colors that nature offers. Celebrate the connection between food and culture, and savor each meal as a moment of gratitude and nourishment.

Above all, remember that your commitment to optimal nutrition is an act of self-love and self-care. It is a lifelong journey that honors and respects your body, mind, and spirit. Be patient, be kind to yourself, and celebrate the progress you make along the way.

As you close this book, let it serve as a guide and a reminder of the transformative power of optimal nutrition. Carry the knowledge and insights you have gained and apply them to your daily life. Embrace the journey, trust the process, and be proud of the steps you take towards your nutritional well-being.

Here's to a lifetime of vibrant health, vitality, and fulfillment through optimal nutrition. You have the power to shape your own destiny, and your choices today will impact your future self. Embrace the commitment, and let optimal nutrition be the foundation upon which you build a life of wellness and flourishing.

Remember, you are capable, you are deserving, and you have everything within you to create a nourishing and fulfilling life. Embrace the journey of optimal nutrition, and let it be the catalyst for unlocking your full potential.

Wishing you a life filled with vibrant health, boundless energy, and the joy of optimal nutrition. Cheers to your lifelong commitment to your nutritional well-being!